How Did That Happen:
Memoirs of a Dyspraxic Diagnostician

By Dr. Linda Buchan

Published by Axia ASD Ltd.

2017

Copyright © 2017 by Dr. Linda Buchan and Axia ASD Limited

Cover Illustrations Copyright © Neve Ellis
Cover design courtesy of Neve Ellis

All rights reserved. This book or any portion thereof may not be reproduced or used in any manner whatsoever without the express written permission of the publisher except for the use of brief quotations in a book review or scholarly journal.

First Printing: 2017

ISBN 978-0-9957661-2-9

Published by Axia ASD Ltd.
Red Hill House
Hope Street
Chester
CH4 8BU

www.axia-asd.co.uk

Dedication

To Albert Atkinson.

The founder of Axia ASD limited

and the love of my life

1955 - 2008

Contents

Dedication 5
Contents 7
Foreword 9
Introduction By Dr Luke Beardon 13
Chapter 1 - Why Write This Book: Beware Of Experts 15
Chapter 2 - Why Diagnose 19
Chapter 3 - How We Diagnose 21
    Dream's Words 23
Chapter 4 - Post Diagnosis/Adjustment To The Diagnosis 31
Chapter 5 - Looking Back At The Past 33
Chapter 6 - The Spiky Profile 35
Chapter 7 - Unwritten Features of Dyspraxia 37
Chapter 8 - Getting Older 39
Chapter 9 - Other Peoples' Perspectives On Dyspraxia 41
    Dyspraxia – From The Outside Looking In 43
Chapter 10 - Cheetahs and Giraffes 49

Appendix 1 - Diagnostic Criteria DSM-5 & ICD-10 51
Appendix 2 - Venn Diagram 55
Appendix 3 - Partnership Model 57
Appendix 4 - Thematic Analysis 59
Appendix 5 - Transition Curve 61
Appendix 6 - Dyspraxia Presentation Conference Slides 63
Appendix 7 - Information Sheet 69

Foreword

I felt the need to establish the original 'intent' and purpose of what a 'Foreword' actually was before putting pen to paper. Forgive me, Dr. Buchan diagnosed my Autism, and as such should perhaps have known better than to entrust such an important task to me, in the knowledge that my approach is not always conventional! That said, my understanding is that a Foreword usually contains interactions between its writer and the book's author in order to give extra context, so here goes...

To have been gifted with the charge of writing the foreword for Dr. Linda Buchan's book *'How Did That Happen: Memoires of a Dyspraxic Diagnostician'* I cannot help but ponder how apropos that question in the title is to my own position this very moment! If I transport my mind back to where I found my Self only five years ago, I had no idea I was about to be diagnosed with AD(H)D, no idea I would then be referred for an Autism diagnosis, and no idea who Axia-ASD or Dr. Buchan were. Neither could I have ever predicted the profound directional change my path through life would take after receiving my diagnosis from Linda.

It is also a privilege to think that in a "book of memories" (if that is what one's 'memoirs' are defined as?) in the relatively short time I have known Linda, I am thought of as 'memorable', and my own reflections of my experience meeting Linda for the first time, as part of a look at an individual's 'pre, per and post' recollections of the Diagnostic Process, have been deemed to contain enough merit to be included within these pages.

I not only felt the obvious emotion of pride when asked if I would write this foreword, but was also somewhat surprised. I would have thought that I was an odd choice, however I know that Linda has an extraordinary insight into my thought patterns and I have great faith in her judgement. Linda has demonstrated an incredible ability to appreciate and accept my idiosyncrasies without moral judgement, and sought to work with (or around) them in order to encourage and assist me in, 'bringing out my best' for the benefit of all. I think, in Linda's terminology, this is called 'The Partnership Model', whilst in my mind, I think of this as '*putting 'Rogerian Theory' into practice'..*

Back in the "old days", when I was diagnosed with a complex neurodevelopmental condition known as Autism Spectrum Disorder, or commonly called Aspergers, the NHS were attempting to assist those of us suffering by offering a number of Post-Diagnostic Support sessions, which, in my case, was six. These were conducted by Linda every few months, and were very much a "life-line" for me. During one of these sessions, at some point I must have mentioned websites, and Linda commented that Carly (Dr. Buchan's proverbial right hand, in some senses) was having some sort of internet issues and I offered to help if I could, in any way. I'm not exactly sure how, but over the years I became more involved with helping Axia evolve their website amongst other things, and at some point, became "part of the team".

I recall expressing to Linda that, touching as it was to feel valued and to be thought of as 'Part of the Team', I have an engrained '*There is no I in team*' mentality and that '*I'm not a team player*' conditioning. If I recall correctly, Linda replied, *"Don't worry, neither am I!"*

In some sense, I am sure this is true: Linda has an integrity of being, which I have witnessed; a willingness to vocalise her thoughts and share her compassion during the post-diagnostic support group meetings which Axia-ASD host, so perhaps Linda is more of a "Leader" than "Team Player", but Dr. Buchan's egalitarian attitude is ever evident, admirable and recognised by many.

I very much resonate with the opening chapter of Linda's book, which begins with a warning: *"Why write this book: Beware of Experts"*. Perhaps less of a warning, and more of an advisory note to the reader that one should be aware of which "tools", "models", and "language" are available to any given "expert".

The next chapter goes on to explain the reason for "Diagnosing" from Linda's perspective, displaying a deep understanding of its purpose, while revealing an idealistic desire in wishing we could evolve past the necessity of this form of medical "labelling", and instead, focus on an individual's strengths and struggles.

After exploring the "why" of diagnosis, the book attempts to explain the "how" of diagnosis (at least in respect of the approach taken by Linda's company, Axia-ASD), going on to address the transition process experienced post diagnosis.

As this book progresses, I find Linda provides an insight into living life with Dyspraxia, a condition I myself display elements of, and the shared commonalities of reprimands, rebukes and reproach Linda experienced seem similar to my own.

And as if to emphasise Dr. Buchan's desire to "co-produce", in the spirit of partnership, those close to Linda have shared their experiences of her dyspraxia.

I do not have the necessary lexical range to discuss the subtlety of psychological and neurological differences conceptually, and therefore am unable to distinguish where my Autism ends and my ADHD begins, or why my dyspraxia, dyslexia and dyscalculia are considered distinct and independent from each other. However, the understanding of my condition, which Linda gave me with her diagnosis, elicited an appreciation and clarity of why my life had been as it had, removing some of the mystery from my history.

And on a personal note, I will be forever grateful to Linda for the opportunities she has bestowed upon me, including encouraging the writing of my book and its publishing, and introducing me to her friend Luke Beardon, an equally awesome individual. Speaking of Dr. Beardon, I do believe his introduction follows this, so thank you for everything Linda, and I'll leave it to Luke to provide a proper piece of writing of a calibre Dr. Buchan deserves!

By: Dream - Voluntary Guest IT Consultant to Axia ASD Ltd. aka Mark G. Etherton

Introduction
By Dr Luke Beardon

I recall very clearly the moment I met Linda - which either says a lot about my memory or, far more likely, the impact that Linda had on me from the moment we met. It was on the first floor of St George's located at Winter Street which is where the Psychology Team was then situated, and I also had an office there. This vibrant character introduced herself in an almost comedic cockney accent, to the extent that I was almost looking over her shoulder to see if she was being accompanied by the Kray twins; her quite frankly lurid purple attire actually seemed to pale compared to her extraordinary strength of presence. I had absolutely no idea just what to make of this person who was insisting that she 'pick my brains' about autism. Bearing in mind, I saw myself as a lowly Project Officer, having this Consultant Clinical Psychologist bringing herself 'down to my level' and ask for *my* advice - this was unheard of. But that's the kind of person Linda was in those days. I am very pleased to say that as far as I can tell, nothing has changed. Linda is, quite simply, one of the humblist people I know. Juxtaposed with an extraordinary intellect which she sometimes hides under a (sincere) veneer of humility and willingness to always listen and learn from others, she makes for a compelling human being with wonderful characteristics and personality. This sounds sycophantic to a ridiculous level; but it's not, it's far more simply just an accurate reflection of Dr Linda Buchan.

I am very pleased to have been a part of what I hope was a genuinely inclusive event for people with all sorts of differing neurotypes, including several with a diagnosis of dyspraxia. It was my wedding. One of the most vivid memories of the day was when there was an announcement that "the dyspraxics are taking over the dance floor" - I'm not sure to this day whether it was a warning, a simple stating of fact, or a triumphant declaration of intent. Whatever, the resulting scenes will last in my memory for a long time - trust me, you had to be there! Words simply cannot describe it, but it was a wonderful part of the day.

I'm so pleased that Linda has taken the time and effort to create these memoirs. And it's equally fantastic that others have shared their experiences within it: it all lends to the richness of the writing, the exploration of the lived experiences, as well as some of the more clinical reflections that Linda brings as a very experienced and highly regarded clinical professional.

It is twenty years (not quite to the day but not far off coincidentally) since I met Linda. I was humbled then by her sincerity, honesty, and self-deprecation; I am just as humbled today, having been asked to introduce her book. If you are very lucky, you will have met Linda in some capacity. If you haven't, don't worry - you've got a brilliant read ahead of you written by her instead.

Luke Beardon, 2017.

Chapter 1
Why Write This Book: Beware Of Experts

People who I trust and respect for many years have been asking me to write a book and I have fiercely resisted this. Primarily, because of my Dyspraxia, I struggle to put my ideas down on paper. I am much better at talking and indeed this book has been written by me making voice memos, which have then been sent to my wonderful colleagues who have typed this and other colleagues have helped by proof reading it and turning it into some form of English.

Some of my resistance to writing a book comes from some reactions I have had to my writing in Academia. I managed to escape such scrutiny for most of my academic life until completing my Doctorate at the University of Sheffield in 2004. I can't remember the date I achieved it, but Carly, my Operational Manager, will remember and will insert this into the book. I often get dates mixed up and confused, again, part of my Dyspraxia.

The external examiners from my Doctorate of Clinical Psychology said at the Viva that the Doctorate could not be put in the public domain as the English was of not a sufficiently high standard and in effect, it had to be re-written – you can imagine how distressed I was. I needed a great deal of support to continue.

At a recent post-diagnostic support group that Axia ASD Ltd run, primarily for people who have been diagnosed with Autism, a member of the group asked me to write a book about Dyspraxia. I think, given my advancing years, that suggestion seemed to resonate more than on previous occasions as I do feel that having had the privilege of meeting lots of people with developmental difference over the years, that I have learnt something about both myself and others, hence the book.

Firstly, what is Dyspraxia, or as some people prefer to call it Developmental Coordination Difficulties. I personally prefer the term Dyspraxia. Perhaps, in part due to my love of the Greek language, but also because I think it describes so much more than the simplistic explanation of coordination difficulties. Dyspraxia is much more than this and I think is better encapsulated from the two Greek words: 'dys', meaning difficulty and 'praxis', meaning action, i,e, difficulty with almost any action, which is certainly how my Dyspraxia impacts on me. The diagnostic criteria, that we as diagnosticians use are shown in Appendix 1 and in order to help the flow of this book, there will be a number of appendices and for some of you reading it; this may not be helpful in having to move from what you are reading, to looking at the Appendix for which I apologise. Feel free not to look at the Appendices.

I self-diagnosed my Dyspraxia subsequent to my wonderful son being diagnosed at the age of 7 with Dyspraxia. This is what we have called the 'Ripple Effect' where I am mindful when I diagnose one family member with Autism or any developmental difference that there is the propensity for other people in the family recognising that they too have developmental difference and indeed, many of my family members do have developmental differences.

Later in his life, my son went on to gain the additional co-morbid co-occurring condition of Dyslexia and it is seen as the rule rather than the exception nowadays, that if you have one developmental difference you are probably going to have another. Therein lies a problem: the minute we try to put people into boxes we fail and with kind permission from DANDO the Venn Diagram shown in Appendix 2, illustrates how people don't fit neatly into boxes, however, the systems around us require, and indeed often demand that we put people into boxes and so diagnosticians should try to put people in the best box that is going to get them the services and support that they need. The only point in gaining a diagnosis is if it is going to make a positive difference to their life. So, therein lies the first problem with trusting experts, that we are only as good as the tools we are provided with and the current knowledge base. Of course, experts are important, however, the way they deliver their expertise is absolutely crucial. The expertise needs to be delivered in "The Partnership Model", see Appendix 3, where the individual and the expert work together in a spirit of mutual respect and mutual trust acknowledging that each person brings their own expertise. So, you are the expert on yourself and parents are the experts on their children, that isn't to say, as parents we don't sometimes get something wrong, but I defy anyone to tell me they know more about my son than I do.

So, given that I have now set myself up in writing this book as some sort of expert, before you close the book and accept that you are the expert on yourself and therefore don't need to read the book, I would like to share some things about my Dyspraxia that I think are not well documented and might be helpful to you or those around you.

Chapter 2
Why Diagnose

There is no point in diagnosing somebody, and indeed, although I have been doing this for most of my professional life, I still fail to see why we have to give people labels in order that they can have their needs met, but I am constantly reminded that without the label people say their needs are not met. I wish we could just describe where people excel and where they struggle but we have to put them into a box and label it. Anyone who tells you it is easy to put people in a box doesn't know what they are talking about (see Venn diagram, Appendix 2). The only reason to diagnose somebody with any Neurodevelopmental condition is if it is going to make a positive difference to their life and we are quite clear when we meet with people that we really do have their meaningful consent; we ask them what difference it would make to their life and we are clear that this is going to be positive.

Chapter 3
How We Diagnose

The way we diagnose at Axia is by engaging in dialogue with individuals, making it clear that the individuals themselves are the "experts" on themselves and parents are the "experts" on their children (Partnership model, see appendix 3). We routinely ask 3 questions:

1. Why have you come to see me today? So that we can all establish why we are in the room together and what we hope to achieve.

2. What difference would a diagnosis make to your life?

3. What is your reaction to the diagnosis? – We have analysed people's responses to these questions using what is called a Thematic Analysis – A number of common themes emerged which are detailed in Appendix 4

4. The assessment process involves initial liaison with the Operational Manager to arrange a mutually convenient appointment. At this stage, an appointment pack is issued to the client containing our detailed developmental history questionnaire which forms part of the assessment. A two hour appointment then takes place with members of our clinical team, using structured and unstructured interviewing, developmental history taking and observations. Subsequent to receiving a verbal diagnosis on the day, a fully detailed assessment report is then released to the client and their GP so that the diagnosis can then be placed on the medical records.

Dream's Words

When Dr. Linda Buchan asked me if I could recite my experience of the diagnostic process and its surrounding events for a section in her 'memoirs', I felt honoured, privileged and humbled to have been thought of. I do not bandy those words about lightly, they are of genuine sentiment.

It is around four years ago now from the date I first met Linda whilst visiting Axia-ASD for my assessment, and as I try to recall my 'mind-space' by re-reading my Specialist Assessment Report and my own 'submission', I find it may perhaps be easier for me to express 'My Story' in the chronological pattern that I recall…

The reason I was referred to Linda in the first place was due to having received a diagnosis of ADHD from Dr. Peter Mason some twelve months prior. It was at the very end of their diagnostic process that Nurse Paula Potter made, what I consider to be, a 'throw away' line as I was leaving the room. That line was *"I knew you had Aspergers as soon as you walked through the door"*. It transpired that this statement was one of those 'life changing lines' one occasionally hears which alters the direction of one's path.

It was very odd to think that something about me and my 'condition' were immediately apparent to another, and so I asked if the diagnosis was in writing. Because of my questioning, my GP was asked to refer me, and I found myself receiving an 'Offer of Specialist Assessment' from Axia-ASD Ltd. to be conducted by Dr. Buchan. This, I believe (from recollection) was accompanied by a Developmental Questionnaire which was to be filled in by my Mother (following consultation with my Sister). Due to my 'character' perhaps, I found my Self wishing to ALSO *'add my two-pence worth'* and respond to the questionnaire. I was in my mid 40s and felt that I had something to say about my life, and so I appear to have written an 'affidavit', 'testimonial' or 'Affirmation of Truth' which I sent to Linda as a private document PURELY for 'Diagnostic Purposes' and "not intended for the Public Record" (these are MY words, verbatim). I also expressed my "Trust Issues", and despite being able to agree to the presence of a trainee psychologist in principle, the quantity of people in a room starts to make me feel uncomfortable when more than 3 (including myself) are gathered.

Some of my memories from the day of assessment are more vivid than others. I remember the horrible levels of adrenaline I experienced when driving over to Chester with my mum, which was the only time I have visited Axia's offices with company for the journey, and haven't gotten terribly confused and even lost when trying to find my way home! Also, the massive amount of relief I felt merely arriving in the car park at Red Hill House in Hope Street. I had time for a smoke before my appointment and thought I had "calmed down" enough following the drive, so mother and I entered the building.

I remember signing in at the front desk, and it not being a long time before being greeted and guided by Carly through what appeared to be a rabbit warren to me. Mother and I were then introduced to Dr. Buchan by Carly who then left we three alone. Despite having visited Axia's offices since, I am trying to recall and envisage my initial visit (as they have multiple rooms now). I couldn't describe with any accuracy what the room looked like bar my perceiving it as *"having good light and good space with a hue of violet"*. I instantly appeared to feel or give a "trust" towards Dr Buchan and please bear in mind that I had stated to her in advance of my suspicious nature and difficulty with this issue! There is something about Linda, which after much thought I still cannot put my finger on, which for me induced an instant trust. I recall my mother trying to "shut me up" because of my babbling and meandering speech, and her concerns with "wasting the doctors time" (I assume), but Linda said something akin to *"don't worry, I'll inform Mark when we've only 15 minutes left"*. Now normally it is ME who is the clock watcher', and I ALSO usually notice others who do the same, however, when Linda said this I had NO idea how long we'd been there or how long I'd been ranting about whatever it was, and remember being impressed of her ability to actually BE PRESENT with my Self and my Mother, but at the same time remain aware of timing.

There are a couple of other 'lines' I remember Linda saying which have stuck with me and need no prompting to recall. One of them was when she turned to my mother and said *"Is he always like this?"* I remember thinking *'Like what?!?'*

My mother replied "yes" to that question, but I think Linda would agree having seen me in numerous circumstances since then, that I displayed a 'relaxed and open nature' which is relatively rare to see (unless you're my Mother!!!). I also distinctly remember being extremely confused when Linda had turned to my mother to 'allay any fears' which mum may have had and said *"don't worry, he's known to the services."* Immediately my mind jumped to the "Police Service" who also use the term "Police Force", however as this was towards the end of the session I did not vocalise my query, but discussed it with mother on our drive home. My mother was able to explain to me that it was more likely to have meant the "National Health Service" (which made much more sense!).

The only other specific comment Dr. Buchan had made, which rings in my head to this day, was whilst I was talking about a film I'd seen called *'A Scanner Darkly'* and Linda made mention of Philip K. Dick, and her knowledge that *'Blade Runner'* was an adaptation of his book *'Do Androids Dream of Electric Sheep?'*

(which was something I did not know, and later wondered why Dr. Buchan would not only have KNOWN it, but also what relevance Philip K. Dick had). It sort of seemed important at the time, however nigh on 4 years later I am still curious, but with all that has occurred since I think it probably trivial in the 'greater scheme of things'.

As I start to re-read the extensive Assessment Report, I find my Self to immediately be a little shocked. In the first section on Social Communication, Dr. Buchan wrote *"Despite Mark not believing my assertions that he was highly intelligent, I was privy to trying to follow some of these complicated and very interesting discussions"*. I perhaps should give this some context as to why I am feeling a certain shock at this minute. Through Axia-ASD, I met Dr. Luke Beardon, who provided or instigated numerous profound experiences for me, the latest being inspiring me to "actually write". A book was born of this, and Linda asserted her wish for Axia to publish it. Because of Linda and Luke's foundational influence in *'Mental Models of Reality'* coming to be, Luke was kind enough to write an Introduction and Linda was gracious enough to write a Foreword. In that Foreword, Dr. Buchan stated that *"I disagree when Dream states he is "not a smart bloke". He is one of the most intelligent people I have met"*. I've known Linda in various capacities and roles now, and I perceive integrity as being one of her most apparent attributes, expressed often irrespective of the 'hat worn'. I still find it extremely difficult to accept this compliment, but feel on some level it must have some merit due to what I perceive as Linda's 'authenticity'. Maybe it is this 'genuine-ness' which others also see.

I feel I should state at this juncture, as I read more of my Assessment Report, that I would not be rereading it had I not been asked to contribute to this section on the diagnostic process for Linda's book. This act is likely to taint my perspective… in fact it is not likely to, it HAS. I appear to have forgotten how much insight into my Self Dr. Buchan had gained from our meeting, how many 'realisations' I appeared to have shared with Linda during the assessment, to then forget, and find my Self thinking them to be only 'recent realisations'. This experience is perhaps a reminder that receiving a diagnosis was as much a beginning for me as it was an end.

At the end of the report were a list of websites and forums which Axia provided, and I recall a feeling of wanting to try to 'Help my Self' by visiting some of them. If I am not mistaken, Dr. Buchan had encouraged me to visit one of the ASD Forums where I may meet "like minded individuals". Unfortunately, my first experience with a well-known (but will go unmentioned) 'community' quickly went South when I was told I was "wrong" by a Moderator of the Forum, and that I must not raise the issue again, with anyone.

At the time, my mind recalled the line from George Orwell's '1984': *"Imagine a boot stamping on a human face forever"*. To be told I was "wrong" when I was CLEARLY and BLATANTLY "right" was not as bad as being told to "stop talking about this topic". I put up no argument, merely apologised and left… and still hold a grudge. Not too long later, I attempted again to join a 'community of like minds', a forum called Asperclick run by Willow Hope. I was immediately contacted by an American chap named Rocco interested in my name (Lord Dream) and whether it was linked to Neil Gaiman. This gentleman is someone whom I really resonate with, and whose artwork I find inspirational. However, his was the only 'friendship' I formed, and it did not take long before I found my Self under attack. I was not aware of the general age gap between my Self and others on the forum, and it turns out 'Millennials' can take offence and lack rationality EVEN IF they are 'on the spectrum'.

I consider myself lucky to have been diagnosed at a time when the NHS were still providing funding for up to six Post-Diagnostic Sessions. Due to my difficulty travelling, these hour sessions were conducted by phone, and felt very much like a 'life line'. In honesty, to be able to have an hour talking to Linda every couple or few months (despite my not liking telephones) was extremely beneficial to me. I have not come across many people in my life who appear to not only have an 'understanding' of me, but also an 'acceptance' of who I am. I felt Dr. Buchan was able to guide me without judgement or dogma (by which, I mean her phrasing of words implied no "You Must").

I have vague recollections of Dr. Buchan inviting me to participate in a 'co-production' group. I remember exchanging emails with Carly as I was not entirely sure what I was being invited to, and although in honesty I never REALLY grasped the purpose of the meeting (apart from something to do with government and funding) I chose to attend. Looking back, I think this was the seed which grew to be Axia's 'Post-Diagnostic Support Group' some months later, which meets every month or so and has provided a plethora of information and support to those who have been diagnosed through Axia ASD. The spirit of co-production is still apparent, we as patients or clients are listened to - what do WE want - and we are heard. Axia's upcoming 2018 conference has been moulded by feedback from the group meetings (at the time of this writing), including its title, content and speakers. I have come across no other companies, institutions or 'those with an obligation' (such as Councils) who appear to achieve such a high level of care and support to so many people as do Axia, and personally I perceive this as being driven by Linda.

Dr. Buchan did ask me to write about the Diagnostic Process, and my apologies if my story contains too much 'Pre' and 'Post' of the 'Process', but as I mentioned, the diagnosis itself was only the start of another journey for me, and due to the stress of the event, my memories are misty. The Assessment Report also contained a Venn diagram and 'Transition Curve' (something else which had slipped from my memory). Looking at it now I feel it is designed to be informative, and yet it contains a "positive bias" in that the curve ends on a high point. I'm not saying that is wrong at all; I'm merely commenting on the fact that the horizontal axis is 'Time', so unless the graph just plateaus out (which in my experience in 4 years has not happened), then one may continue to expect and experience vicissitudes in the 'Proces' as we progress.

I can't really express in words how grateful I feel towards Dr. Buchan and Axia for the support they have shown towards me. I still consider my Self a 'patient' and will not cease claiming *"Dr. Buchan is my psychologist"* (unless instructed otherwise!), despite now also appearing to play other roles, even becoming considered as "Part of the Axia Team" much to my astonishment. In fact, I very much resonate with the title of this book *"How did that happen?"* Not a question I can answer, but I am very glad that 'whatever it was' did!!!

Chapter 4
Post Diagnosis/Adjustment to The Diagnosis

Even for people coming along, positive that they have self-identified that they have a particular Neurological condition, the adjustment process is often much longer, more complicated and perhaps more painful than we realise; the attached Transition Curve, (see appendix 5) is useful. We explain that you may have a range of emotional reactions, or indeed none and that those around you will be going through the same adjustment process, but may be at different points in the course. This can lead to conflict and confusion, for example, if somebody is in denial and somebody else is in the search for meaning stage.

Reflecting back on the past has been something I have done subsequent to my self-diagnosis and has helped to make sense of many of my experiences, but also in some ways, I have looked back on that young child who was punished for things that they couldn't help, with a sense of sadness for that individual. The fact that I still have such acute memories of many of those experiences that are documented in this book, obviously reveals the importance of them and it is perhaps only through undergoing therapy at various points in my life that I have been able to accommodate those; not remain bitter and twisted about them or indeed angry or blaming those people who perhaps often did things in innocence and ignorance. It saddens me that today, despite an enormous knowledge base available that, in particular schools, continue to punish children for things they cannot help and that can have serious implications for their mental health, so any of you reading this that are parents, I would urge you to protect your children from this, to reassure them that their developmental difference is a positive one and it brings many strengths.

Chapter 5
Looking Back at The Past

I would like to share some of those experiences with you, not just to make me feel better, and certainly not for you to feel sorry for me, but to illustrate the following: it is very difficult growing up being made to feel foolish, stupid, lazy and that it's all your fault. Clearly the fact I still need to write about it means it stays with one for a very long time. When you feel like this, it only exacerbates the developmental differences.

I have many memories at school, for example in Domestic Science (shows how old I am, probably called Food Technology now). I was very good at theory and indeed I remember one time, getting over 90% in the theory and the Domestic Science teacher throwing down the results saying "you can't cook a thing". Similarly, with needlework, we weren't allowed to wear our games skirts until we had not only hemmed and stitched them, but also embroidered our initials on them. I tried in vain to do this and I was the only child in the playground that did not have a games skirt in games, but was made to do that in my underwear. I remember one Friday, sneaking it out of school and taking it to my Auntie, who was a very good machinist and embroiderer and bringing it back on Monday, much to the bemusement and astonishment of the teachers, who never found out what had gone on. PE at school was horrendous. I was always hurting myself, was never picked to be part of any teams and in country dancing, I never had a partner. I do love dancing, although my son describes my dancing as looking like a "constipated albatross", but can only dance in my own way, on my own.

I often got told off by my parents for losing money, getting lost, not finding my way back from places. Even now, I can get lost coming out of lifts in hotels. I find bruises on my body that I have no idea where they came from. When staying in hotels, when the bed height is different from what I am used to, I often fall out of bed. I had a very interesting experience at a University presentation, where I not only poured water all over the table, but the plate of sandwiches I was trying to carry. Along with carrying a cup of water, which was very wobbly, one of the sandwiches fell off the plate on to the floor and I trod on it. I was then left with the dilemma of, do I eat the sandwiches, including the one that I had trodden on, or do I sit at the table and not eat anything; I anxiously sat there deciding which would look the least strange option. I could go on and on but I think this gives a flavour of what I have experienced.

Chapter 6
The Spiky Profile

The spiky profile that you see in people with developmental difference means that they are often punished for things that they cannot do.

What do I mean by spiky profile?

People with developmental difference excel in some areas but struggle in others and people often say 'surely if you can do this you can do that'. There is no surely about it: if we could do it why on earth wouldn't we? When people accuse us, and talk to us about this, they often think we are lazy, not motivated or putting it on. Please don't criticise us, we are doing a very good job of it ourselves. Many people have been shocked when I say I can't drive, I then go on to say I would in fact be a dangerous driver and they try to reassure me by saying that they are certain I would be able to pass my test. They may well be right, that I could pass my test, however, I know that I would be a dangerous driver as I could not coordinate the different components that need to be seen in a good driver. There is no surely about it - I would kill people. I have never sat behind a steering wheel and never intend to, so you can all be reassured by this. However, many people with Dyspraxia make good drivers. It is really important not to generalise.

Chapter 7
Unwritten Features of Dyspraxia

- The Dyspraxic Choke.

- Sneezing

- Blowing Your Nose

- Constipation and going to the toilet (triard)

- Incontinence

There are some excellent books written about Dyspraxia, 'Caged in Chaos' by Victoria Biggs and 'Living with Dyspraxia' by Mary Colley, and also 'You're So Clumsy Charley' by Jane Binnion and other books from 'Your Stories Matter' and some references made to some unusual or some un-written features about Dyspraxia, given that Dyspraxia can affect any muscle groupings. The focus tends to be on arms and legs and so on, however, my experience and others self-report is that there are other parts of the body that can be dramatically affected, for example, what I call the Dyspraxic choke. Now swallowing is quite a complex process and the choke can happen even when not eating or drinking, there is also some suggestion that people with Dyspraxia may produce excess saliva which was certainly my case while I was growing up. I also can't eat anything without drinking, I am very anxious if I go somewhere and food is served without some form of liquid. The Dyspraxic choke for me, at its worst, means I need help from others, for example, slapping me on the back as it becomes difficult to breathe. When I sneeze, it is with such ferocity that it can be alarming to others, it's like an explosion. It also took me and others I know, quite a long time to be able blow our noses - I can't seem to coordinate all the components needed. People find this very hard to comprehend. I have always had bowel problems, again I can't seem to coordinate all the muscles in the right way. I realise it must have been a problem for me from a very young age as I used to call "poo" triard, I thought that is what it was called, it's only much later in life I realise that's because, when I was sitting on the potty, my parents used to say to me "try hard" as I was clearly failing to defecate. Continence again, is something that is rarely spoken about. My clinical experience is that particularly for nocturnal enuresis, the traditional ways, such as using alarm systems, do not work. I recommend that the children carry on with pull-up pants for as long as they need to, the pressure is taken off them and their parents. It seems it resolves itself, in almost all cases, by puberty, perhaps as a result of hormonal changes, but I have no research evidence to back this up. Merely my observations. Where it does not resolve itself, I have seen Botox used effectively.

Chapter 8
Getting Older

Dyspraxia doesn't disappear as you get older. I have learnt situations I need to avoid without feeling guilty about that. I suppose, with many of us, as we get older we become more comfortable with who we are and less concerned about what other people think. I have also come to a greater understanding of what my spiky profile looks like and try to embrace what I am good at rather than focusing on what I can't do.

1. Don't "beat yourself up" for things you can't help. If you were in a wheelchair, you wouldn't say "I just need to try harder and then I will be able to get up and walk". Just because people can't see your Dyspraxia or indeed on occasion they can, doesn't mean you don't have it.

2. Surround yourself by people who don't judge you, who embrace your difference and value your strengths. People judging you just makes you struggle more and exacerbates our developmental differences.

3. As well as surrounding yourself by people who don't judge, surround yourself with people who are willing to help.

4. Everybody needs a Carly (see next chapter)

Chapter 9
Other Peoples' Perspectives on Dyspraxia

In the spirit of partnership, I have also asked others to write their chapters on how they perceive my Dyspraxia and what they would like to share about their experiences.

Following on from Chapter 8, everybody needs a Carly, here is her chapter.

Dyspraxia – From the Outside Looking In

I first met Linda over 8 years ago whilst working within the Sheffield Asperger Syndrome Service. At the age of 27, I had never heard of Dyspraxia and so when I was informed of Linda's diagnosis and that due to this she required additional administrative support, I was intrigued to say the least. Not wishing to appear ignorant, I turned to the internet to try and research what this strange sounding word was and what was ultimately required of me in order to provide the best possible administrative support.

I then went into work and plucked up the courage to ask Linda some questions about her Dyspraxia and I found this to be invaluable and the start of our longstanding relationship. We were able to have an open and honest discussion about the areas in which Linda struggles with and how I could adapt the administrative support accordingly so that we complemented each other.

In the early days of working with Linda, I realised that talking was the best strategy as handwriting was difficult to read. Typing was even more difficult (I realised this without even having to ask when I saw how Linda used the office telephone, punching the numbers in with her knuckles rather than her finger tips) and so this is where I really began to understand Linda's thought processes.

The dictation received for reports to type were very different to the ones I had done previously and so in the beginning I used to listen to the entire dictation before actually doing anything so I could grasp an understanding of what was needed, listen to the instructions, process the information given to me and then listen all over again and know which order to do them.

I think to ask anyone with Dyspraxia to follow a structure or template can be quite restrictive and totally unnecessary. What does it matter in which order you do something as long as the end result is the same? I have found throughout my many years of working with Linda that the best ideas and strategies come when we start talking about one topic and somehow end up on a completely whole other subject! I often say that I think Linda's (and Calvin's) brains are constantly working overtime and to try and prevent this would be unfair on them and everyone else.

For me personally, I think Dyspraxia can manifest itself differently in individuals and depends on a number of factors and therefore it is hard to generalise. Within this chapter, I am hoping that I portray Linda's Dyspraxia adequately. For example, Linda herself has stated earlier in the book that she finds it difficult to put her ideas down on to paper whereas she can speak extremely eloquently and articulately. Other people with Dyspraxia, however, (and it is not my intention to make a general stereotype comment), I feel, struggle to actually form the words of what to say whilst their brain and mind knows the answer it is just too difficult to speak them. I think this can also often be visually seen where the mind is working on forming an answer but the words struggle to come out of the mouth. I think each individual over time can develop the best method of communication for them, however unique that may be.

I've learnt many things about various neurodevelopmental differences throughout my time with Linda and the complexity of the conditions is forever changing and evolving. For example, having witnessed the Dyspraxic choke on many occasions, this used to, at first, really frighten me whereas now I know Linda needs me to pat her on the back as soon as she gives me the indicator, a small (or hard) tap is given and the evening continues. However, without that understanding or acknowledgement of this difficulty the outcome of an evening could be a whole different one!

There are small things we, as neurotypicals, can do such as making sure there is a glass of water nearby whenever eating, napkins are also close by for any spillages that may occur, handrails or a gentle arm held whilst walking up or down stairs but most of all not blaming or being judgemental for the areas they may have difficulties with. Sometimes hotels do look really confusing and knowing which way to turn to or which floor to get off does not have to even be an issue but what I have found is that providing that small amount of support allows Linda (and others) to concentrate on their skills instead of weaknesses.

My role in working with Linda is to adapt my working style to accommodate Linda's needs. I provide support to Linda with both personal and professional tasks in organising travel, accommodation, diary management, hair appointments, birthday cards. You name it, I will do it so that Linda can focus on doing what she does best because after all, Buchan definitely does know Best!

Dr Amandip Bahia:

Linda was the first person I met with Dyspraxia, and in fact, I had never even heard of it until she told me, let alone knew what it was. Linda was my tutor when training as a Clinical Psychologist, and soon after I completed a six month placement with her. My first impressions of THE Linda Buchan... well, she seems lovely, definitely knows her stuff and had already told me she would push me to work hard. Linda explained that there were certain things that were very difficult for her: map reading, putting keys in locks, typing etc, were some of the more obvious ones, but I had no idea about the complexities of this condition. My first thoughts were, oh so you are a bit clumsy and can't drive... no big deal! It would have been easy to minimalise the breadth and scale of daily difficulties that can occur as part of this difference, you can't always see it, so it can be hard to understand,

One of the many things I love about Linda, however, is her openness: no question is too silly, too obvious - she is happy to talk about the differences she has, which was great for my curious mind. I was intrigued at how her mind/body worked differently to my own, and some of the anomalies that existed too! It also made me learn about some of the coping strategies which were second nature to Linda, however, fascinated me.

After I qualified, Linda and I worked together in a building that had a very windy staircase. I knew Linda had struggled with stairs and through my work in a Neuro-developmental Disorders Service, I was aware that this was a common difficulty. However, one particular Friday, Linda followed me down the stairs whilst we chatted, and I was struck with the ease of her navigation at the same time as talking to me... so of course I asked her. Linda had a strategy to follow my legs down the stairs, something that was easier on a day when I was wearing a skirt so she could see my legs.

I have (with other friends and colleagues) been asking/nagging/persuading Linda to write this book for some time, her candidness at talking about her personal journey, coupled with her professional insights make her mind something that I think should be shared with as many people as possible. I have been fortunate to have worked for her for a number of years, but I would love for her personal journey to be shared with as many people as possible. We have a saying in the Axia family: Buchan knows best. She hates it! And whilst she wouldn't possibly let me say she is an expert who knows all, I think she knows so much that this book should be read by anyone who is curious about Dyspraxia!

Chapter 10
Cheetahs and Giraffes

I very much wanted my son to contribute to this book as he has Dyspraxia and Dyslexia and for many months I asked him how he might contribute to the book; whilst he sincerely wanted to make a contribution, it just wasn't happening. I then came up with the idea that perhaps he could use the presentation he did at our Dyspraxia Conference in October 2014, an excellent presentation which was well received (see Appendix 6) along with the other presentations on Dyspraxia that were made at the conference. I then made the suggestion that he could turn the power point presentation into a chapter, perhaps using voice memos to do so. Despite support from his supervisor and our administrative team agreeing to help him, again it wasn't happening.

I thought long and hard about what that might be about and was somewhat annoyed as it was holding up the publication of the book, but then I realised that, despite being someone with Dyspraxia and despite being a diagnostician of Dyspraxia, I was doing to my own son, what people do to those of us with a spiky profile. Perhaps we accept that they might have done something exceptional in one area, in my son's case, he had done a brilliant presentation, however, it is never good enough and we want them to do something else, that we know they are going to struggle with, so I wanted my son to write a chapter for a book, which, given Dyspraxia and Dyslexia is probably something that he is going to struggle with enormously.

I've called this chapter Cheetahs and Giraffes. So, we all acknowledge that giraffes are very good at reaching up to leaves on tall trees and we all acknowledge that cheetahs are very good at running. However, we also acknowledge that cheetahs cannot reach up and pick up leaves from the tops of trees and that giraffes are probably not that good at running. What we tend to do with people with spiky profiles is we say to the giraffes, we don't want you to spend your time doing something you are good at, reaching up and eating leaves at the tops of trees, rather, we want you to spend your time practicing being able to run faster. We say to the cheetahs, we don't want you to spend your time running fast because you are already good at that, we want you to learn how to better reach the tops of trees and eat the leaves. Clearly this is soul destroying and demoralising. So, I apologise here and now, to my son, for waiting months for him to write a chapter for my book, but rather I shall let his presentation suffice and I urge you to look in Appendix 6.

Finally, as part of the research for this book and thinking about the past, particularly thinking about the partnership model, I was brought back to my partner Albert, to whom this book is dedicated and he was the founder of Axia back in 1998.

We co-wrote an article, which was published in the Australian Journal of Grief and Bereavement (2000) where we wrote about our work with a young girl with Rett Disorder and I was struck by the fact that much of that article was saying the same as this book, the importance of working in partnership, the importance of not judging and above all, the importance of people listening to individuals as they are the only ones who truly know what their lives are like.

Appendix 1 - Diagnostic Criteria DSM-5 & ICD-10

The DSM-5 Diagnostic Criteria for Developmental Co-Ordination Disorder (American Psychiatric Association, 2013)

A. Motor performance that is substantially below expected levels, given the person's chronologic age and previous opportunities for skill acquisition. The poor motor performance may manifest as coordination problems, poor balance, clumsiness, dropping or bumping into things; marked delays in achieving developmental motor milestones (e.g., walking, crawling, sitting) or in the acquisition of basic motor skills (e.g., catching, throwing, kicking, running, jumping, hopping, cutting, colouring, printing, writing).

B. The disturbance in Criterion A, without accommodations, significantly and persistently interferes with activities of daily living or academic achievement.

C. Onset of symptoms is in the early developmental period.

D. The motor skill deficits are not better explained by intellectual disability (intellectual development disorder) or visual impairment and are not attributable to a neurological condition affecting movement (e.g., cerebral palsy, muscular dystrophy, degenerative disorder).

Dyspraxia

(ICD-10 Classification of Specific developmental disorder of motor function)
F82

The ICD-10 Classification of Specific developmental disorder of motor function,

The main feature of this disorder is a serious impairment in the development of motor coordination that is not solely explicable in terms of general intellectual retardation or of any specific congenital or acquired neurological disorder (other than the one that may be implicit in the coordination abnormality). It is usual for the motor clumsiness to be associated with some degree of impaired performance on visuo-spatial cognitive tasks.

Diagnostic Guidelines

The child's motor coordination, on fine or gross motor tasks, should be significantly below the level expected on the basis of his or her age and general intelligence. This is best assessed on the basis of an individually administered, standardised test of fine and gross motor coordination. The difficulties in co-ordination should have been present since early in development (i.e. they should not constitute an acquired deficit), and they should not be a direct result of any defects of vision or hearing or of any diagnosable neurological disorder.

The extent to which the disorder mainly involves fine or gross motor coordination varies, and the particular pattern of motor disabilities varies with age. Developmental motor milestones may be delayed and there may be some associated speech difficulties (especially involving articulation). The young child may be awkward in general gait, being slow to learn to run, hop, and go up and down stairs. There is likely to be difficulty learning to tie shoe laces, to fasten and unfasten buttons, and to throw and catch balls. The child may be generally clumsy in fine and/or gross movements – tending to drop things, to stumble, to bump into obstacles, and to have poor handwriting. Drawing skills are usually poor, and children with this disorder are often poor at jigsaw puzzles, using constructional toys, building models, ball games, and drawing and understanding maps.

Scholastic difficulties occur in some children and may occasionally be severe; in some cases there are associated socio-emotional-behavioural problems, but little is known of their frequency or characteristics.

There is no diagnosable neurological disorder (such as cerebral palsy or muscular dystrophy). In some cases, however, there is a history of perinatal complications, such as very low birth weight or markedly premature birth.

The clumsy child syndrome has often been diagnosed as "minimal brain dysfunction", but this term is not recommended as it has so many different and contradictory meanings.

Includes: Clumsy child syndrome
Developmental coordination disorder
Developmental dyspraxia

Excludes: Abnormalities of gait and mobility (R26.-)
Lack of coordination (R27.-) secondary to either mental retardation (F70-F79) or some specific diagnosable neurological disorder (G00-G99)

Appendix 2 - Venn Diagram

The Make-up of Neuro-Diversity

This is a document for discussion. Concentrating mainly on the difficulties of those with neuro-diversity. It must however, be pointed out that many people with neuro-diversity are excellent at maths, co-ordination, reading etc. We are people of extremes.

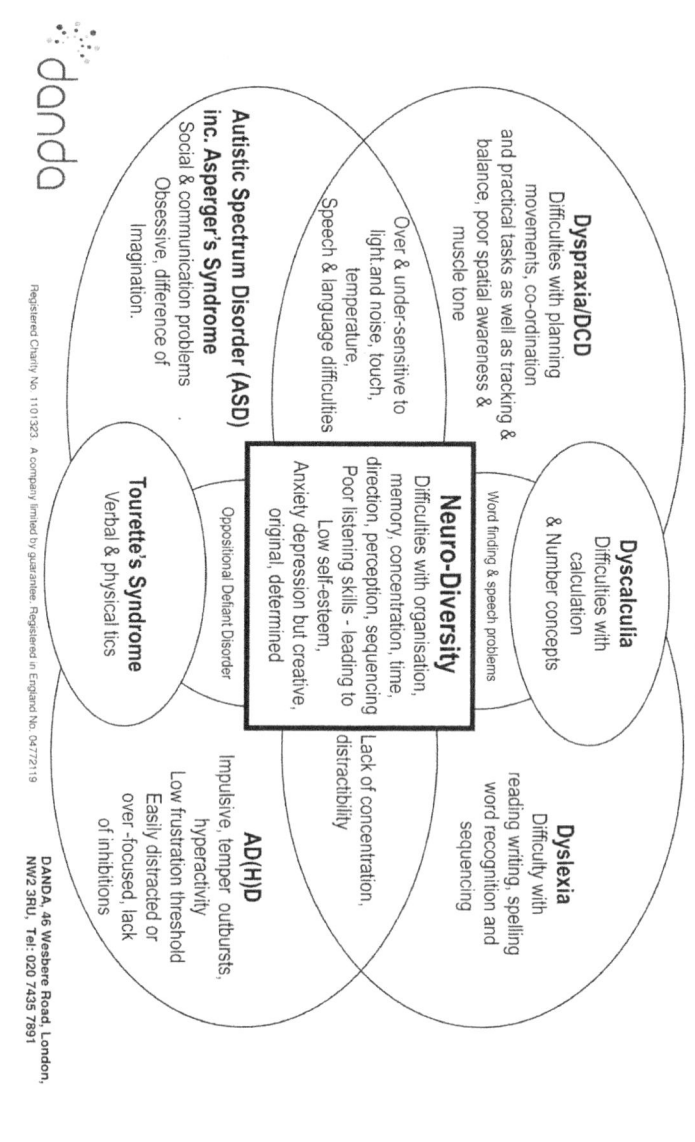

danda

Dyspraxia/DCD
Difficulties with planning movements, co-ordination and practical tasks as well as tracking & balance, poor spatial awareness & muscle tone

Autistic Spectrum Disorder (ASD) inc. Asperger's Syndrome
Social & communication problems Obsessive, difference of Imagination.

Over & under-sensitive to light and noise, touch, temperature.
Speech & language difficulties

Tourette's Syndrome
Verbal & physical tics

Opposition Defiant Disorder

Neuro-Diversity
Difficulties with organisation, memory, concentration, time, direction, perception, sequencing Poor listening skills - leading to Low self-esteem,
Anxiety depression but creative, original, determined

Word finding & speech problems

Dyscalculia
Difficulties with calculation & Number concepts

Lack of concentration, distractibility

Dyslexia
Difficulty with reading writing, spelling word recognition and sequencing

AD(H)D
Impulsive, temper outbursts, hyperactivity
Low frustration threshold
Easily distracted or over-focused, lack of inhibitions

Registered Charity No 1101323. A company limited by guarantee. Registered in England No. 04772119

DANDA, 46 Wesbere Road, London, NW2 3RU, Tel: 020 7435 7891

Appendix 3 - Partnership Model

www.cpcs.org.uk

The Partnership Model is a process of helping. It has many theoretical underpinnings, including the work of George Kelly in terms of Personal Construct Theory, Carl Rogers – Person Centred counselling and Gerard Egan – Problem solving. It acknowledges that people are the "experts" on themselves and we need work closely together, sharing power, but being led by the parent or the individual, recognising complementary expertise, agreeing aims in the spirit of mutual respect, openness and honesty. The essential qualities of the helper are respect, unconditional positive regard, genuineness, empathy, humility, quiet enthusiasm, personal integrity. The skills needed are the ability to actively listen, to prompt and explore, to respond empathically, to summarise, to enable change and to problem solve. With gratitude to Professor Hilton Davis.

Appendix 4 - Thematic Analysis

Themes

- Upon final analysis, 7 common themes were found among the data. The quotes from the theme "severity of condition" were found to sit better within the 'loss & regret' and the 'unsure of diagnosis' themes:

  - 1) Understanding of Self (n=24)
  - 2) Closure & Relief (n=30)
  - 3) Loss & Regret (n=4)
  - 4) Emotional (n=3)
  - 5) Hope for the Future (n=7)
  - 6) Conformation of Suspicions (n=12)
  - 7) Unsure of Diagnosis (n=17)

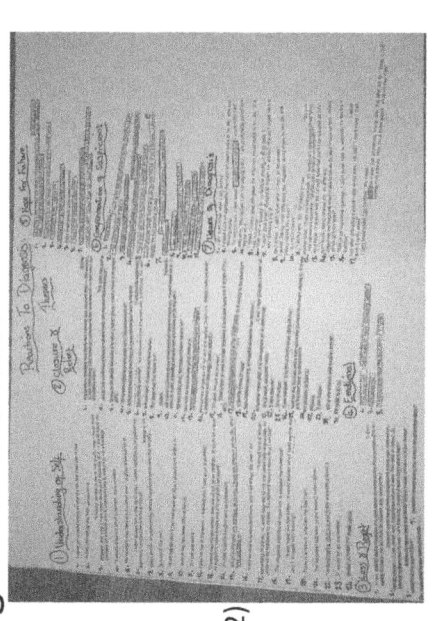

Appendix 5 - Transition Curve

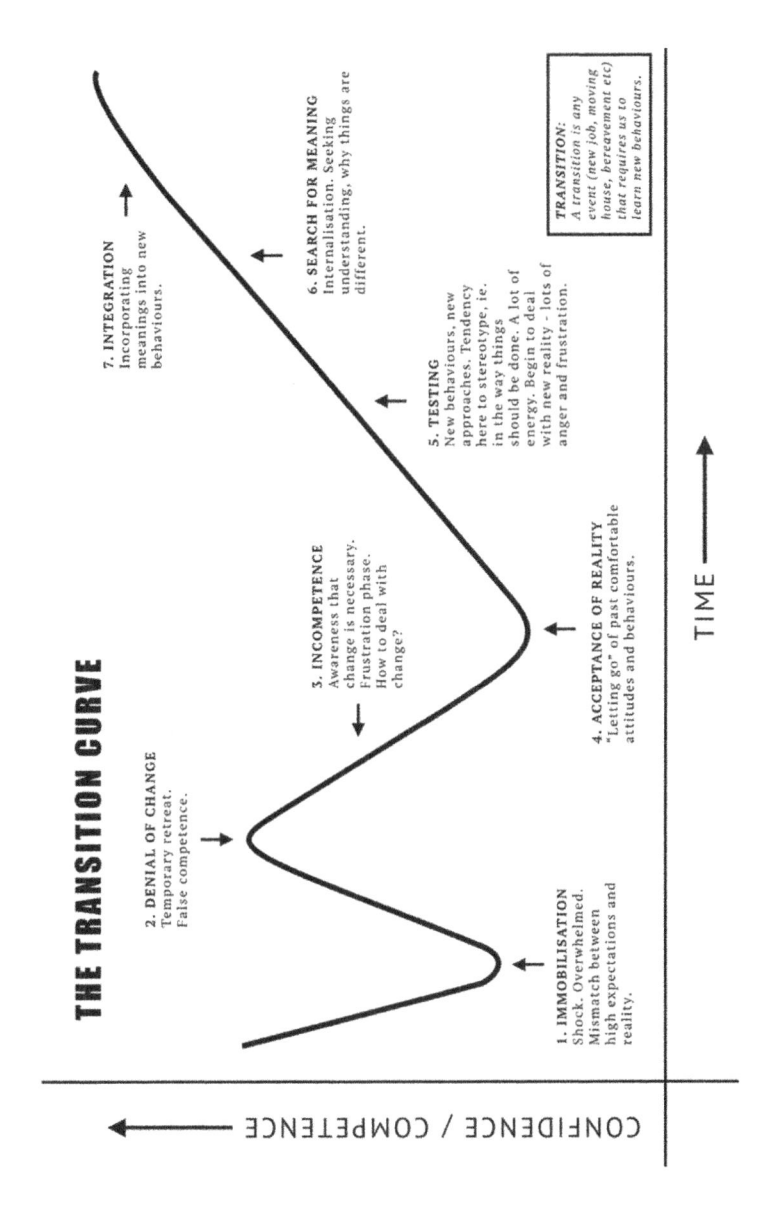

THE TRANSITION CURVE

1. IMMOBILISATION
Shock. Overwhelmed. Mismatch between high expectations and reality.

2. DENIAL OF CHANGE
Temporary retreat. False competence.

3. INCOMPETENCE
Awareness that change is necessary. Frustration phase. How to deal with change?

4. ACCEPTANCE OF REALITY
"Letting go" of past comfortable attitudes and behaviours.

5. TESTING
New behaviours, new approaches. Tendency here to stereotype, ie. in the way things should be done. A lot of energy. Begin to deal with new reality - lots of anger and frustration.

6. SEARCH FOR MEANING
Internalisation. Seeking understanding, why things are different.

7. INTEGRATION
Incorporating meanings into new behaviours.

TRANSITION: *A transition is any event (new job, moving house, bereavement etc) that requires us to learn new behaviours.*

Axes: CONFIDENCE / COMPETENCE (vertical), TIME (horizontal)

Appendix 6 - Dyspraxia Presentation Conference Slides

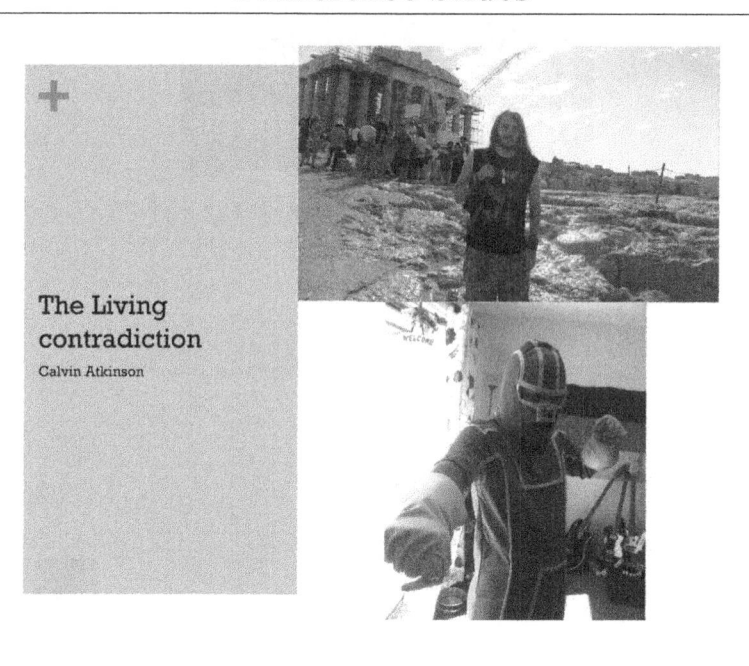

The Living contradiction

Calvin Atkinson

+introduction

Calvin Atkinson

- Chef
- Consultant on youth and Nerd Culture for AXIA ASD Limted
- Film reviewer for Axia Film society
- Diagnosed with Dyslexia and Dyspraxia

File photo

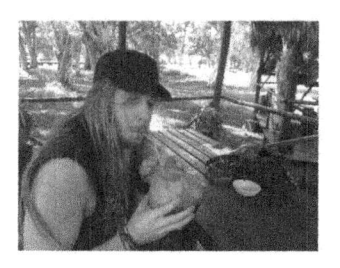

YOU ARE MADE OF STUPID!

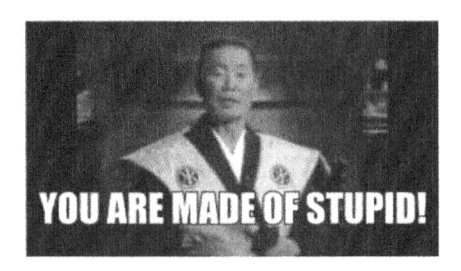

General public view of dyspraxia

Clumsy
Weird
"not really disabled"

How do I/We respond

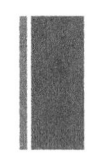

- https://www.youtube.com/watch?feature=player_detailpage&v=MV0sK65PyVI
- https://www.youtube.com/watch?v=WrjwaqZfjIY
- https://www.youtube.com/watch?v=PetqKh7lr8g

inspiration

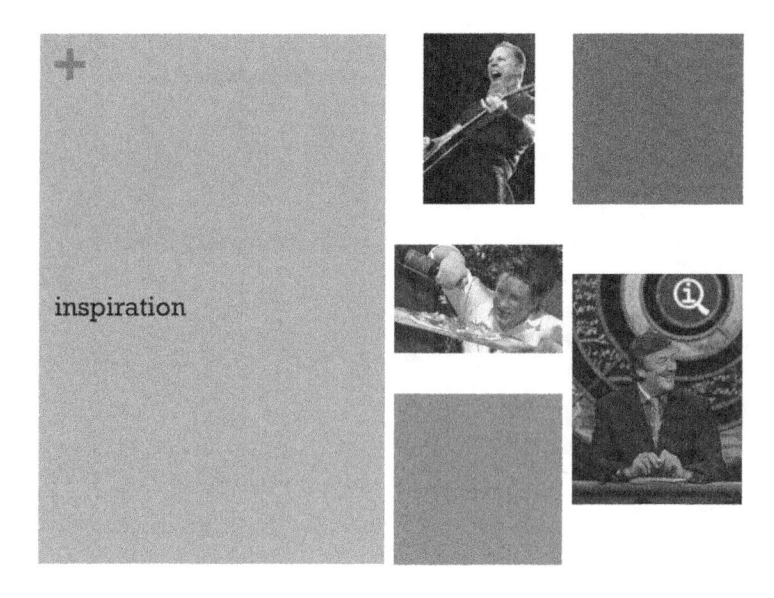

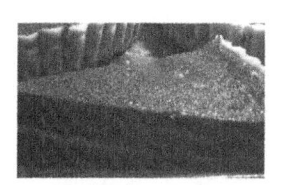

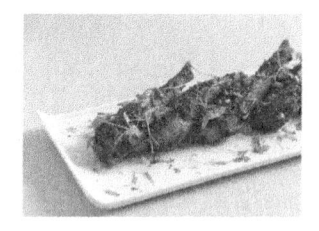

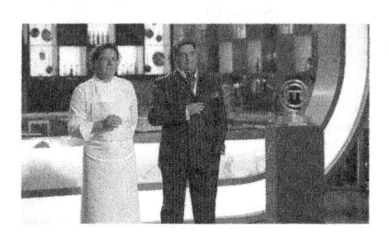

+ Dyspraxia for chefs
Marco Pierre White

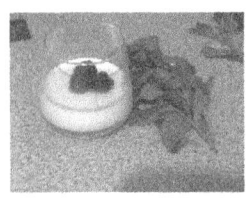

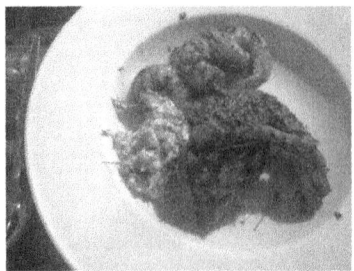

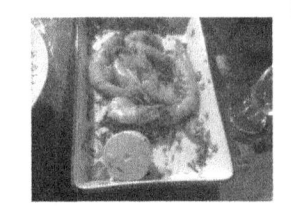

Dyspraxia for chefs

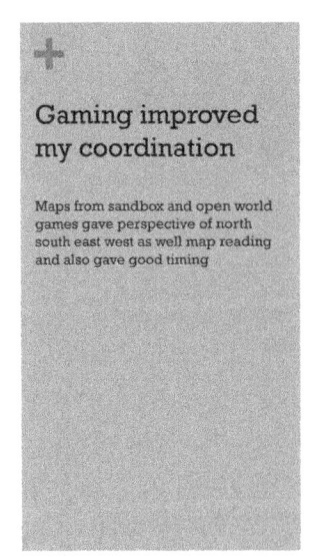

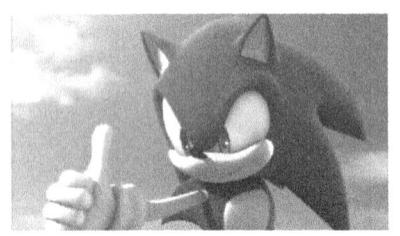

Gaming improved my coordination

Maps from sandbox and open world games gave perspective of north south east west as well map reading and also gave good timing

A dyslexic guy that wanted to read

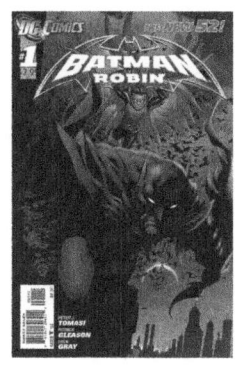

- Grew my love comics
- Great works till accessible
- audiobooks

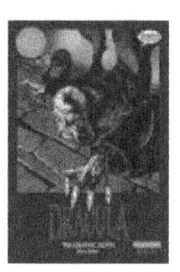

Disability is only one part of the story

- It doesn't define what we can and can't do
- It may limit us but it doesn't prevent us
- https://www.youtube.com/watch?v=vhe3vSe-mmw

How Did That Happen:
Memoirs of a Dyspraxic Diagnostician

Appendix 7 – Information Sheet

Information Sheet - DYSPRAXIA

Useful Website Addresses for Information via the Internet

www.nhs.uk/carersdirect - NHS Choices Website for Carers providing free, confidential information and advice

http://www.dyspraxiafoundation.org.uk/ - Offer support, information and advice regarding Dyspraxia

http://livingsensationally.blogspot.co.uk/ - For Adults with sensory sensitivities

http://www.funkygerbilpress.com

Useful Telephone Numbers

The Carers Direct Hotline – 0808 8020202

Book References - *Some of these may be more or less relevant. There are many books available, however,*

detailed below are ones we would recommend. We regularly review books on our website www.axia-asd.co.uk.

1. Caged in Chaos: A Dyspraxic guide to breaking free Updated Edition by Victoria Biggs, published by Jessica Kingsley.

2. Living with Dyspraxia: A Guide for adults with developmental Dyspraxia by Mary Colley published by Jessica Kingsley in 2006.

3. Life through a Kaleidoscope: Experiences of Scotopic Sensitivity Syndrome - Memoirs of visual fragmentation by Paul Isaacs and James Billett published by Chipmunka in 2013.

4. The Dyspraxic Learner: Strategies for Success by Alison Patrick published by Jessica Kingsley

5. You're So Clumsy Charley by Jane Binnion published in 2013.

6. You Can't Do That by Sue Wood published by Funky Gerbil Press.

7. Kids in the Syndrome mix of ADHD, LD, Autism Spectrum, Tourette's, Anxiety and More by Martin Kutscher.

8. I'll tell you why I can't wear those clothes: Talking about tactile defensiveness by Noreen O'Sullivan published by Jessica Kingsley in 2014.

9. Creative, Successful, Dyslexic. 23 High Achievers Share Their Stories by Margaret Rooke published by Jessica Kingsley.